SHAKEN, NOT STIRRED:

Living with Parkinson's Disease

Larry Linton

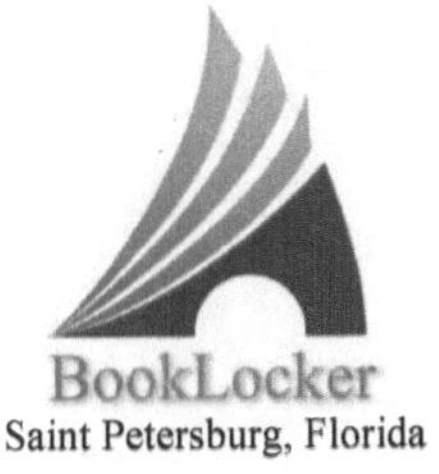

BookLocker

Saint Petersburg, Florida

ISBN: 978-1-64718-551-0

Published by BookLocker.com, Inc., St. Petersburg, Florida.

Printed on acid-free paper.

BookLocker.com, Inc.
2020

First Edition

Disclaimer

This book details the author's personal experiences with and opinions about Parkinson's Disease. The author is not a healthcare provider.

The author and publisher are providing this book and its contents on an "as is" basis and make no representations or warranties of any kind with respect to this book or its contents. The author and publisher disclaim all such representations and warranties, including for example warranties of merchantability and healthcare for a particular purpose. In addition, the author and publisher do not represent or warrant that the information accessible via this book is accurate, complete, or current.

The statements made about products and services have not been evaluated by the U.S. Food and Drug Administration. They are not intended to diagnose, treat, cure, or prevent any condition or disease. Please consult with your own physician or healthcare specialist regarding the suggestions and recommendations made in this book.

Except as specifically stated in this book, neither the author or publisher, nor any authors, contributors, or other representatives will be liable for damages arising out of or in connection with the use of this book. This is a comprehensive limitation of liability that applies to all damages of any kind, including (without limitation) compensatory; direct, indirect or consequential damages; loss of data, income or profit; loss of or damage to property and claims of third parties.

You understand that this book is not intended as a substitute for consultation with a licensed healthcare practitioner, such as your physician. Before you begin any healthcare program, or change your lifestyle in any way, you will consult your physician or other licensed healthcare practitioner to ensure that you are in good health and that the examples contained in this book will not harm you.

This book provides content related to topics physical and/or mental health issues. As such, use of this book implies your acceptance of this disclaimer.

Table of Contents

"I am thankful for my struggle, because without it, I wouldn't have stumbled upon my strength."

- Alexandra Elle

Introduction

In 1969, Elizabeth Kubler-Ross wrote in her book, "On Death and Dying" that grief could be divided into five stages: denial, anger, bargaining, depression, and acceptance. Although originally devised for people who were terminally ill, the stages have been adapted for other experiences with loss, too.

Forty-three years later, in 2012, confronted with a life changing diagnosis of Parkinson's disease at the age of 49, I went through the same stages. Each stage was experienced, but not necessarily in order. Sometimes, I felt like I went through all five stages in one day. Other times, my day would start with depression, but as the day progressed, I became frustrated, and angered. Some days, I could not actually define what stage I was experiencing. I just knew that I was not myself.

You may have picked up this book because you have recently been diagnosed and struggling to cope with such an unexpected life changing event. You may be the caregiver who has now been, unexpectedly, shouldered with the burden of the condition, too. You are feeling overwhelmed with all the incessant questions flooding into your head, but you don't have any answers. You lie in bed fretting about your career, your home, the well being of your family.

This book purposefully avoids subjects like the possible causes and risk factors of Parkinson's disease, the pharmacology of the disease, the various stages of the condition and its progression. Instead, the book essentially starts with the premise and a fundamental question: you've got it, now what?

To answer that question, and the underlying reason for writing this book, is to share with you my own experiences through the same stages of grief. More importantly however, this book gives you a look into my life before my diagnosis, the dark days that followed "the day of," but then, more importantly, how I managed to start to enjoy a life that is, in many respects, more rewarding, fulfilling and meaningful AFTER my diagnosis, than before. My sincere hope is that it helps get you to the same stage far sooner than me, so that you can regain control and continue to enjoy a life that is worth living, and to do so for many years to come. Parkinson's disease does not control or define me. I want the same for you.

CHAPTER ONE
Diagnosis Delivered

*"The diagnosis can be done in
about two lines. It doesn't
engage anybody"*

- David Foster Wallace

"Parkinson's disease is a chronic and progressive neurodegenerative disorder for which there is no cure."

I read that on an information pamphlet in the waiting room at my first appointment with a neurologist. All I could focus on were the words: Chronic. Progressive. No cure.

Three years before the appointment, I became conscious of a slight, but continuous, twitching of my small finger of my right hand. It was the first thing that I noticed every morning when I woke up, lying in bed after the alarm clock went off. Then, a few months later, my right leg started dragging, and I noticed that I was walking with a sort of flat, dropped foot. I didn't have a natural heel-to-toe gait, it was more like a slapping motion. I saw my GP to discuss these issues but, in his opinion, I was anxious. I was too young to have Parkinson's disease. It was all in my head. I came up with excuses: too much coffee was causing the twitching in my hand. My dragging leg was a result of too much running, I pretended to myself.

I saw a Chinese herbalist and he told me I should live near water and prescribed something to drink that tasted as bad as it looked. Sessions at a physiotherapist, hypnotist, acupuncturist, and herbalist followed. Three years later I had developed a resting tremor in the whole of my right hand. I could hardly walk, let alone run.

Even years before, I noticed tremors in others: I watched the HBO series "Real Sports with Bryant Gumbel" interview with Freddie Roach (the trainer of the boxer Manny Pacquiao) talking about how he confronted living with Parkinson's disease. I focused on his right hand. My hand had a similar tremor. Before coaching, he had been a professional boxer and took blows to the head. That's why he got Parkinson's disease, I convinced myself to think.

I saw Muhammad Ali light the Olympic Flame during the opening ceremony of the 1996 Atlanta Games, his left arm shaking uncontrollably as he did so. He was in the advanced stages of his fight against Parkinson's disease, a fight that he unfortunately lost in 2016. I rationalized that, again, it must have been all those years of taking blows to his head that caused him to get the disease.

Then, of course, I saw Michael J. Fox. I have always liked Michael J. Fox. On my first trip to the United States, and after seeing him in "Back to the Future," I had to find those same red striped, white leather Nike sneakers, as well as a pair of Original 501 Levi's that his character, "Marty McFly," wore in the movie. Later, watching him on "Family Ties," I tried to adopt the same preppy look of "Alex P. Keaton" as a young law student at the University of the Witwatersrand in Johannesburg, South Africa, right down to the same tanned executive briefcase that he used in the show.

Years later, when he announced that he had Parkinson's disease, I was sad for him.

Little did I know, I would have something more in common with him besides sneakers and jeans. He told a similar story about a resting tremor in his left hand as the earliest symptom and the start of his journey with Parkinson's disease. He was 30 years old at the time, working on "Doc Hollywood," his fifth film in three years. He was a busy actor, not a professional boxer! I was neither, but I had the same tremor.

The appointment with the neurologist comprised of a full medical history including the checking of my vitals, like blood pressure, pulse check, heartbeat, lungs and the usual "prod and poke" around the abdomen. The examination quickly progressed to a brief neurological examination and observation for balance, coordination, tapping and extending the fingers, and the writing of a sentence. All of this lasted 30 minutes before I heard it officially: "It's my opinion that you have Adult Onset Parkinson's disease."

But what I really heard was: Chronic. Progressive. No cure.

So, just like that, after 3 years and 30 minutes, I finally had a diagnosis. At long last, I knew what I had, and didn't have to bother about trying to get an opinion from another list of health providers. The doctor recommended one drug to start (Mirapex) to be taken three times a day and wanted to see me again in a month. That was it.

Chronic. Progressive. No cure.

No mention was made of those three topics. Nor did he address his history of treating patients with Parkinson's disease. Nothing on his overall treatment philosophy. It was all very clinical, and unemotional.

Waiting to finalize my next appointment with the receptionist, I noticed that the waiting room had filled up. I looked at some of the faces and I wondered how many would be getting the same news that I had just received. How many other lives would be impacted and forever changed from that day forward? What does it all mean? What happens now, today and tomorrow? I had no answers. My only focus was on the words: Chronic. Progressive. No cure.

Returning to the office, and to the pile of files on my desk, no longer seemed important. I needed to be at home. When I got home, I poured myself a whiskey – it was 5:00 PM somewhere! I booted up my laptop and typed into Google and YouTube, "Parkinson's disease." I was traumatized at what I read and watched. I had no terms of reference or any understanding of what I was reading or seeing – "freezing," "dyskinesias," "dystonia," "dopamine agonists" were words that were suddenly added to my vocabulary, but with no real understanding of what they meant.

The images that I saw terrified me. People sitting in chairs, shaking uncontrollably, some walking with flailing arms and legs, some with expressionless faces, others drooling. Was I looking at my future self? How was I going to live with an old person's disease at the age of 49? How was I going to provide for my family as the principal wage earner?

That day was the start of another traumatic period of my life.

CHAPTER TWO
Adversity From The Start

"There is no education like adversity."

– Benjamin Disraeli

My very first childhood memory was a traumatic one, too. It was the day my father died. I was 6 years old. He was only 45. Close my eyes, and I am back in our house in Bloemfontein, South Africa on that very day – February 18, 1969. I can remember staring through a crack in his bedroom door, seeing him lying on his bed. He is surrounded by a few people who I don't recognize. There is a lot of activity and blurred motion around the room. I can't see his face. At some point, I am ushered to the living room to sit on the sofa. I can sense that something different is happening. It doesn't feel like a regular day.

The next vision is seeing my father being wheeled down the corridor on a gurney and out of the house. I would never see him again. My mother's face is stricken with pain. I feel stuck to the sofa. I can't jump off it. I realize, at that moment and at such a young age, that my life from that day on would never again be the same.

I learned about my father from my older siblings, and my mother. After finishing high school, at the age of 19, he joined the South African Air Force and was based in Italy as a bomber pilot during the Second World War, under the command of the British forces. My brother spent many hours putting together a thick binder that detailed his postings, and copies of the actual sorties that he flew. After the war he qualified as a pharmacist, owned two pharmacies in Bloemfontein, and married my mother in 1950.

I was told that my mother and father were on stage as amateur performers. They were also on a radio game show and won a new fridge! From time to time growing up, I used to play the tape recording of the show because you can hear my mom interacting with the host of the show, but more importantly, I got to hear my father's voice, too. It was literally a sound bite, but I took comfort in hearing his own voice.

Apparently, he was a heavy smoker and suffered two heart attacks before his third, and last, in 1969. It must have been awfully hard on my brother and sister. They were teenagers at the time and that event would profoundly reshape their lives, too. My brother assumed a lot of the responsibility for the well being of our family at a noticeably young age and he continues to do so in many respects, even today, while enjoying his new role as grandfather to five. My sister had a tougher time adapting to her new reality and has faced some challenging events in her own life, but she has survived them with a formidable strength of character and great determination.

I was too young to feel the loss of my father. Any void was filled by my mother, and my siblings. I always felt loved, and still do. I may not have been rich in material terms, but I felt rich in many other ways: deep and unbreakable bonds that kept our family together, as well as the strong, personal friendships that have endured for more than 45 years, despite miles and time apart.

Being an amateur performer, my mom played the piano and sang. I obviously inherited some of her "performance genes" because I developed a love for drumming at a very young age. I never took a drumming lesson. I had a good "ear" and was able to identify the rhythm and beat of a song very easily. I banged my mother's furniture to pieces with my drumsticks, until she bought me a small practice pad. A second-hand drum set followed, but that didn't last long. My mother received complaints from the landlord on the noise that I was producing in a two-bedroom apartment. I had to return to the practice pad, but in my mind, I was surrounded by a ten drum set with a double bass and sixteen cymbals.

My mother dragged me to a lot of movies, mostly musicals, and loved to listen to jazz on the radio. At a young age, I was introduced to "The Rat Pack," Ella Fitzgerald and "Satchmo," to name a few.

Being the youngest by at least ten years, I spent more time with my mother. From an early age, I got to understand her and know how hard it must have been for her to be shouldered with the burden of bringing up three children on her own. My mother passed away from Non-Hodgkin's

Lymphoma at the age of 63. I kept her voice mail message for years after her passing, so that I could hear her voice again.

I met my future wife, Melissa, when I was 17 and going into my last year of high school. She was 15 and going into Grade 8. We were both in Cape Town on vacation and met through common friends. After that summer vacation, we continued seeing each other when we returned to Johannesburg. Her life was the opposite of mine. She went to a private school and was a dedicated student. She got good grades. Melissa had a very stable family life living with her parents, a younger sister, and grandparents in a house with a pool, on the better side of town. For the first few years, I had to address her parents as "Mr." and "Mrs." Visits to their house were by their invitation only. A few years into my relationship with Melissa, I could then call them by their first names.

Our relationship continued through university and we were the first couple of our friends to be engaged and married. I was 23 and she was 21.

We were also one of the first couples to leave South Africa. During the 1980s, South Africa was in turmoil. At times, the country was under a state of emergency which gave the security forces extraordinary powers of arrest, detention without trial, and a wide range of interrogation methods. The courts lacked judicial independence under those circumstances and the media was controlled by the state. Nelson Mandela was still serving a life sentence as a convicted "terrorist." However, the country faced sanctions and economic ramifications as international businesses, celebrities and other governments pressured South Africa to end the "separate, but equal" regime.

Once my law studies were complete, I faced two years of compulsory national service. I could no longer defer reporting for duty after five years of university studies and one year of working as a "trainee lawyer."

Newly admitted lawyers were based at the Phalaborwa Commando Unit, located approximately 500 kilometres, north-east from Johannesburg and very close to the entrance of the Kruger National Park. The main reason for being based in Phalaborwa was to complete three months of infantry training and then be assigned to prosecuting the army recruits who were claiming status as "conscientious objector," or who were being court marshaled for going AWOL (absent without leave).

Quite simply, I didn't see my future in South Africa. So, instead, with the understanding from our respective families, we left for Auckland, New Zealand in 1989.

That same year there was finally a shift in South African politics. A more liberal Prime Minister was elected on the basis that it was time to negotiate to end apartheid. In February 1990, he lifted the ban on the African National Congress and other opposition groups and released Nelson Mandela from prison. In 1994, Nelson Mandela became the president of South Africa.

By then, Melissa and I were on the move again, this time to Toronto, Canada with our son Daniel, born in 1992. A daughter, Jenna, followed in 1994.

We were the epitome of the more traditional family. I was steadily progressing through my career as a corporate immigration lawyer, commuting to and from the office two hours a day and making it home just in time to bathe and tuck our kids into bed. Melissa was working full-time as a personal trainer, but arranged her schedule to pick up the kids from school, help them with their homework, get them to and from their extra mural activities, and generally running our home with military precision. Weekends were filled with dance recitals, soccer tournaments, enjoying each other's company, visiting friends and extended family, and laughing a lot. We were lucky to enjoy many memorable vacations in Florida, Mexico, the Dominican Republic and Saint Martin.

My drumming was confined to banging out a beat to a song on the steering wheel in my car. I was a weekend runner, limited in distance and time. I hardly broke a sweat during those runs.

Like all long-term relationships, there were times when we faced ups and downs and the usual challenges. As our kids grew up, our needs changed, like deciding whether to take another job, deciding to sell our first home and where to buy. At times, we disagreed with each other, but we managed to get to a consensus and return to our "normal" everyday routine.

The early death of my father brought into sharp focus my own mortality. Knowing that there was a clear genetic link, I was convinced that avoiding heart disease would be my life's health challenge.

Boy was I wrong! Instead, a diagnosis of Parkinson's disease, at the age of 49, presented a much bigger surprise and greater challenge. How would the relationship with my children change? How would I be perceived by them? A failure? Would they be embarrassed by me if they saw me shaking uncontrollably? Would they still take my advice? What about my relationship with my wife? Would she still love me? How would our roles change? What had I done to get this? Would I be able to continue working?

CHAPTER THREE
Living a Lie

"No lie never reaches old age."

- Sophacles

I had absolutely no idea how to even start to formulate answers to those questions. So, I took what I thought was the best course of action. I decided to deny what I had. I started to come up with fresh excuses. I'd ride a bike instead. It was better for your knees. I was in denial and became very adept with creative excuses.

The medication as originally prescribed wasn't working. My hand tremor was still very much continuous, so the neurologist added an additional drug (Sinemet) when I met him for my second appointment. For a few weeks after that, I began to feel nauseated and dizzy and, when I tried to discuss it with him, he seemed to get impatient with me to the point of saying, "Mr. Linton, either you take the medication or you don't, it's your choice." That wasn't the response I was looking for at only my second meeting. Faced with a chronic, progressive condition I didn't expect sympathy from him, but I was looking for a better partnership in what was going to be a long professional relationship.

I started looking for another neurologist.

In the meantime, I became more conscious of my hand tremor, so I shoved my hand into the pocket of my pants, or would clasp my hands together, or even sit on my hand. I would try and stay seated at my desk in the office for as long as possible, so that I didn't have to walk around. I routinely asked one of my team members to fetch the lunch that I had ordered and ate it at my desk. I even tried to limit my washroom breaks during the day, so that I would avoid being seen dragging my leg down the corridor.

Sustaining that routine for the first year or so after my diagnosis became exhausting and emotionally draining. My body started reacting negatively to the pressure. My anxiety increased dramatically, and the tremor in my hand intensified. I became an insomniac. I hardly slept. When I was asked why I looked so exhausted, I had another excuse. There was a late overtime game that I just had to finish watching.

And then, the start of panic attacks. The very first happened while sitting on the train commuting into the office. I was reading the morning's newspaper. Out of nowhere, my heart started racing, my head started spinning. I felt the urgent need to jump up and out of my seat. I started sweating. I lowered the newspaper and felt many eyes on me. My thoughts became frantic and irrational. I was having a heart attack, just like my dad. I thought about hitting the emergency strip but noticed that we were already pulling into the station. I stumbled out of the train, made it out of the station, and jumped into a taxi to get back home. I must have looked bad, because the taxi driver kept glancing at me and from time to time, kept asking if everything was okay. Of course, I was okay; it was just something I ate for breakfast that was not agreeing with me. Another excuse!

These attacks continued and could start anywhere, anytime: in the car, in a movie theater, while eating out with friends or family. But I noticed that they didn't occur all that much at home. So, for much of the first two years I became a recluse.

I made it into the office but withdrew further away from my team. I declined team meetings and pretended that I was too busy. I declined client events, too. All I wanted to do was to get back to the safety of my home, and to my sofa. The sofa became my "safety zone." I watched my family from that sofa, like I had watched my mother all those years before, when my father died.

Away from the office, and socially on weekends, things were not much better. I used to have panic attacks in the parking lot waiting to join friends for dinner. I had a client stuck at the border and had to deal with the immigration authorities. More excuses. My wife got used to excuses, and even came up with some new ones on my behalf.

I discussed these issues with my GP. He prescribed an anti-anxiety drug. My routine was to take an anti-anxiety pill in the morning, my Parkinson's "cocktail" three times a day, and then a sleeping pill at night. I was knocked out cold on the sofa for the night and felt so "foggy" during the day that I couldn't think straight.

The panic attacks became less frequent, but I could not clear my head and started withdrawing from my wife and kids. I became less talkative and spent the weekends on the sofa staring blankly at the television. I couldn't even make it to the dinner table to engage in conversation with them. My friends gave up on calling me. I never returned their calls in any case. My wife started joining them alone on the weekends. My kids lost interest in me, too. Even our dog, Becky, gave up jumping onto the sofa to join me. I ate and slept on the sofa. Leaving my home to get into the office became torturous. I was "foggy" pretty much the whole day and kept myself behind closed doors. I hated my life.

I discussed this also with my GP and he prescribed more medication. This time, anti-depressants. So, within two years of my diagnosis I was anxious, depressed, couldn't sleep, and had Parkinson's disease. All at the age of 51 – what a life!

CHAPTER FOUR
Finding My Rhythm

"One day you'll tell your story of how you've overcome
what you are going through now,

and it will become part of someone
else's survival guide."

- Unknown

It was another typical Saturday night. I was alone, sitting on my sofa again. This time, like the sudden start of a panic attack, I felt an intense wave of emotion rush through me. I became teary. I started crying. I couldn't stop. I started heaving and wailing like a baby. Two years of pent up emotion fueled by denial, anger, anxiety and depression came gushing out of me like a tsunami. I thought again of my father. I recalled the pained look on my mother's face on the day he died. I cried. The more I thought about my family, the more I cried. The more I thought about the future, the more I cried. The more I cried, the more I cried. At some point, I reached a point of exhaustion.

And then -- utter calm and peace. I had not lost my father. I was a 51-year-old with Parkinson's disease. I was still a father, a husband, a friend. I still had a good career.

My life still had meaning. I still had hopes and dreams for myself and my family.

I had to get off the sofa. I did.

Right there and then, I went upstairs and retrieved my running clothes from the back of my wardrobe. I put on my running shoes and went downstairs into the basement. On and around the treadmill were some discarded household items and a layer of dust. I cleared those away, and gave the console a quick wipe down, and then fired it up. I started walking. I ignored my dragging foot. I held on to the treadmill, forcing myself to keep going. The important thing was that I was moving forward, literally.

Melissa was pleased to see my exercise gear in the laundry basket that night. I kept adding to it.

Every morning, before leaving for the office, I would walk on the treadmill for ten minutes. I started noticing that my right leg no longer dragged as much, while on it, and off it. I returned to a more natural gait. I persevered and started adding a minute of jogging after a ten-minute walk. As the weeks rolled into months, I started reducing my walking, and increased the running, first to 20 minutes, non-stop, then 30 minutes with a walk, then 45 running, and then 60 minutes, nonstop!

I took my running outside. I was out on the road early in the morning before sunrise. I didn't listen to music. I preferred to hear my feet hitting the road, with equal stride and balanced sound. I no longer sounded like a galloping mule, with a limp. I loved the freedom of those early morning runs. On the weekends, I steadily increased my distances. My head was no longer "foggy." My mind was calm, even while panting up another hill. After my run, I felt energized and my legs felt fatigued. If my right leg dragged, I no longer had to lie. It was from too much running. By the time I got home from work I was tired, and fell asleep very quickly, in bed, not on the sofa.

Much has been written about the benefits of incorporating a regular exercise routine to deal with the motor symptoms of Parkinson's disease. A recent study[1] has concluded that high intensity treadmill exercise may be feasible and prescribed safely for patients with Parkinson's disease. The study recommends that the aerobic exercise should be intense enough, to the point of panting, but not too intense to the point of exhaustion. Typically, this means exercising within the range of 65-85% age adjusted

---

[1] Schenkman et al. *Effect of High-Intensity Treadmill Exercise on Motor Symptoms in Patients With De Novo Parkinson's Disease: A Phase 2 Randomized Clinical Trial.* JAMA Neurology, 2018; 75(2):219-226

heart rate maximum (that is, 220 minus your age), or at between 13-18 on the Borg Scale of perceived exertion.

Another study[2] has found that exercise potentially increases functional circuitry in the brain. Increased dopamine is released in that part of the brain called the caudate which is related to cognitive function, which may explain why many exercise programs show improvement to cognitive function.

Bottom line is that exercise is beneficial for Parkinson's disease. But, a word of

---

[2] Abbruzzese et al. Rehabilitation for Parkinson's disease: Current outlook and future challanges. Parkinsonism & Related Disorders. 2016 Jan. 22 Suppl 1: S60-4

caution, don't expect to train at that high threshold from the start. It took a few months to get to get up to 60 minutes of running non-stop. It's a case of building to that intensity. Your lungs and knees will thank you. Commit to 3 times a week to start, on days, and at times when you are "on" (For me, that is usually an hour after taking my medication, and before eating breakfast). Adopt a "10-30-10" routine, at a comfortable heart rate intensity:

1. Warm up for 10 minutes, with brisk walking.

2. Spend the next 30 minutes at the designated heart rate.

3. Cool down for 10 minutes, again with brisk walking.

Build the routine gradually to the desired 65-85%/13-18 intensity range over a few weeks, or even months, by increasing your speed, increasing the incline (if on a treadmill), and alternating between lower and higher intensities.

Overall, the type of exercise that you choose must depend on your symptoms, fitness level, and overall health. Walking, swimming, water aerobics, yoga, and tai chi are some alternative suggestions to consider. The most important point is to keep moving.

I have kept up my running, and slowly increased my running distance over the years to the point of completing three half-marathons in five years.

Oh, and I haven't taken a sleeping pill in years.

Based on the great results I was having with my running, I decided to return to drumming with more determination. I hoped that it could help with the tremor in my hand. I purchased an entry level electronic drum set that I could play with headphones, more quietly. I wish I could have had that in my mother's apartment in South Africa. I turned to hand drumming as well, and my collection of instruments expanded to bongos, congas, timbales and incorporated other accessories like blocks, claves and — of course — cowbells. You gotta have more cowbells!

The more I played, the less my hand twitched, and the fluidity in my arms increased dramatically, overall. As with my running, I persevered. I took some lessons online, then took Latin hand drumming lessons in person and, once I felt comfortable with my new drumming patterns, I ventured out to "open mics" around town. Those efforts paid off, and I was invited to join two bands and play with one of them in the internationally renowned "Beaches

International Jazz Festival." My mother would have been proud!

Turns out that the brains of musicians are wired differently. Brain scanning studies have shown:

- Increased neural connectivity during music participation and even music listening [3]

- Musicians have bigger[4] brains

---

[3] Alluri et al. Large-scale brain networks emerge from dynamic processing of musical timbre, key, and rhythm. NeuroImage 59(4), Februray 15, 2012, 3677-3689

[4] Schlaug et al. Increased Corpus Callosum Size in Musicians. Neuropsychologia, 33(8), pp. 1047-1055, 1995

- Music participation causes structural changes in motor, auditory processing and visual-spatial areas of the brain [5]

Recently, a narrative literature review [6] of 27 articles found that music therapy has beneficial effects for the treatment of motor and non-motor symptoms, and quality of life for persons with Parkinson's disease. It concludes on a very positive note (no pun, intended!), that the use of music as a

---

[5] Schlaug G. Chapter 3-Musicians and music making as a model for the study of brain plasticity. Progress in Brain Research, vol. 217, 2015. pp.37-55

[6] Garcia-Casares N. Music Therapy in Parkinson's Disease. JAMDA, December 2018 Vol. 19, Issue 12, pp: 1054-1062

therapeutic tool, combined with conventional therapies, should be considered.

But it's not just about playing music. It's about being exposed to it and enjoying everything about it. Other modes of music participation and benefits include:

- Dancing to music, improving gait and balance.

- Playing an instrument (my personal favourite), improving coordination and timing.

- Singing, improving loudness.

- Listening to music, improving mood and quality of life.

- Mental singing, reducing freezing.

Up to that point, I was focusing on the physicality of my condition. I was enjoying the euphoric "runner's high" while running and getting lost in the musicality of my drumming. But, both of those activities were undertaken while in motion.

I started wondering if there were any benefits that could be achieved by doing nothing. My research led me to the practice of mindfulness.

Fundamentally, the practice of mindfulness starts with your breathing. Breathing is the only human act that we can do both consciously and unconsciously, as well as voluntary and involuntary. Our breathing is controlled by two different sets of muscles and nerves, each operating independently. Almost all of us spend most of our lives breathing unconsciously.

Unconscious breathing is ineffective, done without purpose or control. On the other hand, deep full breaths into the belly engage the muscles of the diaphragm and lungs, which in turn stimulates blood circulation. Circulation of blood is the prime physical nourisher of the body and brain, and the mechanism for cellular waste disposal.

It gets better. Deep, controlled, rhythmic breathing helps keep the body healthy because it shifts the body away from the fight-or-flight mode. By focusing on our breath, we allow our somatic nervous system to reprogram the autonomic nervous system. My day always starts with a 15-minute-deep breathing exercise. Every day.

A recent study[7] acknowledged the significant distress impacting the physical, emotional and social functioning in Parkinson's disease patients and their caregivers. The study concluded that mindfulness has a role to play as a protective

---

[7] *Hicks A et al. The role of dispositional mindfulness in a stress-health pathway among Parkinson's disease patients and caregiving partners. Qual Life Res 2019 Oct;28(10):2705-2716*

factor against the psychosocial burdens imposed on all of us with the disease.

The question that I had when I started this new morning routine was, how I could be sure that my breathing was deep enough? I felt relaxed, and my heart rate slowed down, but how could I be sure that I was truly benefiting from the exercise? It's far easier if you are running or exercising. You know when you are panting up another hill. I was more skeptical when sitting on the floor, cross-legged and breathing deeply. I did some more research and was pleased with what I found.

My research led me to "Muse." Muse is a portable EEG device that looks like a high-tech headband that you wear on your forehead, anchored by your ears. It uses advanced signal processing to interpret your mental activity to help guide you with your breathing. When your mind is calm and settled, you hear peaceful weather. As your focus drifts, you hear stormy weather that cues you to bring your attention back to your breath. It connects to your mobile device via Bluetooth. Once connected, you simply start the Muse Meditation app, put on your headphones, and close your eyes. Once your session is complete, you can review your results and track your progress.

I was impressed. It was extremely easy to use, accurate and I have used it consistently for a few years now. I only have one suggestion – rebrand the product as "Muse – Meditation for Dummies." Disclaimer: No trademark infringement intended.

I also use "The Breathing App." It's a free app that I have found highly effective to calm my breathing, which in turn slows down my heart rate and quiets my mind.

I have learned that mindfulness is about controlling your thoughts. When you can master your thoughts, you can control your reaction to them, and be able to focus your attention. Ultimately, it's about training yourself to focus your attention on the present, dispense with ruminating on the past, and avoid getting anxious about the future.

But, it's more than just controlling your thoughts. In his book[8], Rasmus Hougaard summarizes the benefits of mindfulness as follows: "Mindfulness training increases the density of grey cells in our cerebral cortex, the part of the brain that thinks rationally and solves problems. Cognitive function improves, resulting in better memory, increased concentration, reduced cognitive rigidity, and faster reaction times. Not

––––––––––––––––––––––––

[8] Hougaard, R et al One Second Ahead 2016, 1st Edition

surprisingly, people who practice mindfulness techniques report an overall increase in quality of life."

Over time, and with earnest practice, I have been able to essentially rewire my whole thought process. I have implemented mindfulness sessions whenever I have needed to: moments before a presentation, planning for an important meeting, or when stuck in traffic. I have become less reactive to negative thoughts. I have stopped feeling sorry for myself. I no longer compare myself to others. I am no longer consumed about what my future life might be.

With a calmer mind, and being grounded in the present, it's easier to find gratitude, too. I start each day with gratitude. I don't get out of bed in the morning until I have thought of at least one thing that I am grateful for. I write it in my journal with a date so that I can recall what I was grateful for on a specific day.

On August 15, 2014, I wrote: "I am grateful that I took the last dose of my anti-depressants."

CHAPTER FIVE
To Disclose or Not to Disclose

*"It is often wise to reveal that which
cannot be concealed for long."*

- Friedrich Schiller

Based on the latest estimates[9], in 2013-2014, approximately 84,000 Canadians aged 40 years and older were living with Parkinson's disease and 10,000 more were newly diagnosed.

---

[9] *Public Health Agency of Canada, using Canadian Chronic Disease Surveillance System data files contributed by provinces and territories, July 2017.*

It is estimated that the number of Canadians living with the disease will double between 2011 and 2031, and that the incidence will increase by 50%. Nearly one million people in the United States, and more than 10 million worldwide are living with Parkinson's disease according to Parkinson's Foundation.[10] It affects both men and women (with men being slightly more susceptible to getting it) and from all ethnic backgrounds. The average age of onset is 60,

---

[10] The Parkinson's Foundation is a US-based national organization established in 2016 through the merger of the National Parkinson Foundation and the Parkinson's Disease Foundation and has offices in Miami and New York City.

but it can affect people as young as 30 or 40.

Being diagnosed at 49, below the average aged onset, brought up more issues to think about, particularly relating to my job: How long would I be able to work? Should I disclose my condition to my employer? How would the disclosure impact my career advancement?

I felt burdened with the following dilemma: Did I have the obligation to disclose my condition? If I did, could I lose my job? Would my career still advance, if I disclosed?

I did not want to rush into my boss's office the day after getting my diagnosis.

But, at the same time, I didn't want to withhold the news until symptoms became more visible and began to affect my performance.

A booklet[11] published by Parkinson Canada estimates over 90% of people with chronic medical conditions live with the condition that is invisible. Also known as a hidden disability, it is a disability that is not immediately obvious to onlookers and may go unnoticed under most conditions and situations. The studies have also shown that if it cannot be seen, and it will likely be

---

[11] Parkinson Canada, *At Ease: A guide to improving accessibility in the workplace and on route for people with invisible disabilities*, 2018

misunderstood, and, ultimately, not accommodated.

If an employee chooses not to disclose their disability, an employer will not have an opportunity to understand those needs and to provide appropriate accommodations. But, unaware of the disability, the employer may come to view the employee unfavourably.

An accommodation is a mutually agreed and implemented plan designed to meet the specific needs of a person with a disability. This plan may include a change to the working location, the number of hours they work, or the way the professional development and training are delivered.

With my symptoms well managed and under control, after three years of my diagnosis, I decided to tell my team first. There was overwhelming support, and the reaction was simply "we knew." I followed that up with a meeting with my immediate boss. I prepared for the meeting from her perspective. I had no intention of telling her the history of the challenges that I had faced getting to the point of good maintenance. All I wanted to convey to her, truthfully, was that my neurologist was pleased with the current maintenance of my symptoms, that the progression of the disease was uncertain and that I had every intention to work for as long as I had always intended.

Of course, my decision to disclose was a very personal one. For me, it brought a further sense of relief and allowed me to continue to be an authentic leader to my team.

From a legal perspective, specifically in Canada, the issues of disabilities in the workplace are complex. There are several legal principles involved that must, in turn, be balanced against others; for example, the duty of an employee to perform their job safely, and the impact that Parkinson's disease (or other disabilities) could have on their safety and the safety of others.

I'm glad I did disclose, because of what I had started to experience in the office.

CHAPTER SIX
Loss of Words

"Much wisdom often goes with fewest words."

- Sophocles

Being at a loss for words - literally - is one of the challenges that I have faced with my condition.

I have been in meetings, and after being asked a question, I have struggled to formulate a quick response; or in a social setting and have failed to find the right words to contribute to the conversation.

Traditionally, as discussed in an online article published[12] in <u>Future Medicine</u>, Parkinson's disease has been classified as a movement disorder. But many people with Parkinson's disease experience slowness in thinking, loss of memory and decreased attention span. Additionally, research over the past two decades has made it clear that multiple communications deficits are associated with the disease, too. These deficits manifest as both difficulties comprehending others and contributing

---

[12] Holtgraves T. Solutions for improving communication with Parkinson's Disease Patients. Future Medicine, published online November 9, 2016

satisfactorily to verbal communication with others.

Recognizing that communication fundamentally involves two parties – the talker and the listener – the author of the article[13] provides techniques for both to adopt.

First, if the conversation involves a complex matter, the conversation partner should try to avoid words with complex meanings grouped in sentences that require working memory to decipher what the

---

[13] Holtgraves, supra

sentence could mean. For example, try and avoid a sentence like the one I just wrote!

Otherwise, I may invoke a memorable line by Denzel Washington in the movie "Philadelphia," by responding: "Now, explain it to me, like I'm a two-year-old."

Secondly, speakers should lump the information they are conveying into smaller units and wait for an acknowledgment before moving on. Thirdly, topics should be clearly defined and fully dealt with before moving onto the next topic.

Over and above comprehension difficulties, Parkinson's disease has also been associated with abnormalities in speech fluency in the form of prolonged pauses and incorrect verb usage. (There may be some in this book, too. Please accept my apology, but I have an excuse!)

One study[14] examined spontaneous language production and found fluency disruption in the form of long-duration silent hesitations. Another study,[15] has concluded that people with Parkinson's disease display a significant impairment on

____

[14] Illes J. Neurolinguistic features of spontaneous language production dissociate three forms of neurodegenerative disease: Alzheimer's, Huntington's, and Parkinson's. Brain Lang. 1989; 37(4):628-642

[15] Henry JD, Crawford JR. Verbal fluency deficits in Parkinson's disease: a meta-analysis. J Int Neuropsychol Soc. 2004;10(04):608-622

measures of both semantic (When words are similar in meaning; for example, fruit, but the word uttered is different – saying "apple," when the intended word is "orange.") and phonetic fluency. (When words sound similar, but don't mean anything similar; for example, saying "free" when intending to say "four" or "fire.")

These are just two studies, of many, that provide considerable evidence [16]for a cluster of specific production deficits including lowered informational content, speech fluency abnormalities, long and

---

[16] *See in: Communication impairment in patients with Parkinson's disease: challenges and solutions - Holtgraves T, Cadle C J. Parkinsonism and Restless Legs Syndrome*

inappropriate pauses, and impaired grammar.

There is better news, however, in other research. In a doctoral research paper[17] the authors examined whether brief meditation training affects cognition and mood when compared to an active control group.

After four sessions of either meditation training or listening to a recorded book, participants with no prior meditation experience were assessed with measures of mood, verbal fluency, visual coding, and

---

[17] *Mindfulness Meditation Improves Cognition - Evidence of Brief Mental Training, published in Consciousness and Cognition, Vol. 19, No.2: pp. 597-605,*

working memory. Both interventions were effective at improving mood, but only brief meditation training reduced fatigue, anxiety, and increased mindfulness.

Moreover, brief mindfulness training significantly improved visuo-spatial processing, working memory, and executive functioning. Their findings suggest that as little as four days of meditation training can enhance the ability to sustain attention; benefits that have previously been reported with long-term meditators.

That's the research. Now to the practice what I have adopted:

First, when put on the spot by a question, I delay responding, even for just one second. I consciously inhale and exhale. I have found that this routine allows my brain to disengage from the natural "fight or flight" hijack allowing my words to catch up to my calmer brain.

Secondly, I ask for the question to be repeated, or say something like, "Before I answer that, I just want to clarify what you are asking...." Again, this gives me time to formulate a response.

When I do respond, I consciously talk slower than I normally would. Besides not being able to formulate the correct words, I tend to speak too quickly, so this technique gives me time to formulate words and more sentences at a steadier pace.

Wherever possible, I respond last. I let others give their point of view first. That gives me the most time to formulate a fuller response and allows for a longer lasting impression.

Lastly, I sometimes don't respond at all. There may be times where a hand gesture, a wink or a pat on the back could convey the same expression non-verbally. There is strength in silence.

CHAPTER SEVEN
You Are What You Eat

"The only way to keep your health is to eat what you don't want, drink what you don't like, and do what you'd rather not."

- Mark Twain

"You are what you eat."

"You can't out train a bad diet."

These quotes are not in my journal. I don't memorize them either. I don't have to. I hear them firsthand. Often. From my own immediate family.

You see, Melissa is a personal trainer. Jenna is a kinesiologist and osteopath. Daniel went into the family business, on his mother's side. He's a personal trainer, too.

I am constantly reminded to focus as much on my diet and nutrition as I do on my exercise routine. Being genetically predisposed to high cholesterol, and with my father's death at the young age of 45 from heart disease, I have always been acutely aware of my own mortality.

But the truth is, living with a chronic progressive disease, for which there is no cure, takes precedence. So, when it comes to food, I cut myself some slack. To me, everything about food is social. The preparation, the cooking, and then sitting down to enjoy the meal with family and friends is more of a social event than the meal itself. I love to engage with family and friends around the table, over a great meal. In the first few years after my diagnosis, I couldn't get off the sofa to sit at the table. I never want to experience that feeling of isolation again.

That said, I'd still like to share some thoughts about diet and nutrition.

In a recent study[18] out of New Zealand, researchers designed a pilot, randomized controlled trial to compare the plausibility, safety, and efficiency of a low-fat, high carbohydrate diet versus a ketogenic diet in a hospital clinic of Parkinson's disease patients. In total, 44 participants commenced the diets: 20 of 22 completed the low-fat diet, while 18 of 22 completed the ketogenic diet over a period of eight weeks.

The study found that it is plausible and safe for Parkinson's disease patients to

---

[18] Mathew C.L. et al. *Low-Fat Versus Ketogenic Diet in Parkinson's Disease: A Pilot Randomized Controlled Trial, Movement Disorders,* 33(8), 2018

maintain a low-fat or ketogenic diet for eight weeks. It noted that both diet groups significantly improved motor and non-motor symptoms, but the ketogenic group showed greater improvements in non-motor symptoms.

The study concluded, with caution, that a ketogenic diet could play a complementary role in the treatment of Parkinson's disease, but due to the preliminary nature of the findings, larger and longer randomized controlled studies are needed before this can be stated with more confidence.

Diet and the medication can impact each other. Parkinson's Foundation [19] notes that levodopa medications, like Sinemet, carbidopa/levodopa extended-release capsule (Rytary) or carbidopa/levodopa/ entacapone (Stalvo) work best on an empty stomach.

Taking the medication close to a protein-rich meal may interfere with the absorption of the drug in the blood stream, causing it to work more slowly or less effectively.

---

[19] https://www.parkinson.org/Living-with-Parkinsons/Managing-Parkinsons/Diet-and-Nutrition

Other recommendations to consider include the following:

- Take the medication with a full glass of water.

- Limit sugar intake, alcohol and caffeine.

- A Mediterranean diet is best – like vegetables, fruits, herbs, beans and whole grains.

- Incorporate some yogurts.

- Adding a vitamin D supplement should be considered.

- The addition of over-the-counter dietary supplements should be discussed first with a pharmacist or other health care professional.

- The levopoda effect is not comprised by protein meals, provided that the carbidopa/levodopa doses are taken at least an hour before or at least two hours after the completion of meals[20]

I do appreciate the fact that my family only has the best of intentions when they remind me of my dietary shortcomings. But, they have come to accept the fact that, from time to time, I will indulge and have a

---

[20] Ahlskog J. E. *Pakinson's Disease Treatment Guide for Physicians.* Oxford Press, 2009, p. 302

second scoop of ice-cream. For me, it's more about enjoying all types of food, but in moderation and limiting my alcohol intake.

CHAPTER EIGHT
Do The Opposite

*"Take the course opposite to custom
and you will always do well."*

- Ashley Madekwe

If I could rewind the clock, there are several things that I would have done differently in an attempt to reduce the roller-coaster ride of emotions that I endured in the early stages of my journey with Parkinson's disease.

It took me ten years to join a support group. But, joining a support group would have given me much needed support, emotionally and mentally, from the start.

As we went around the table, each attendee introduced themselves and briefly outlined their journey with Parkinson's disease. One was diagnosed only a month before, some within the last year, a couple of others weren't taking medication at all, some were seeing a naturopath, another had gone through Deep Brain Stimulation, and one was being scheduled for that procedure. We all had the opportunity to engage and learn from each other. I found it therapeutic, as we shared experiences on various topics like medication, the importance of diet and exercise, the importance of rest, the benefits of mindfulness, and the importance of allowing yourself to grieve. Then, with the symptoms well managed and under control, to reintroduce laughter and joy into living a full life with Parkinson's disease.

From time to time, I glanced over to the "newbie" and at times she was very emotional and tearful. But she was there, a month into her journey, and that was the crucial difference. At the end of the session, she was smiling and interacting more confidently with the others. She learned firsthand that Parkinson's disease affects everyone differently, and that the direction and progress will be varied and as different as each person. She learned in two hours what it had taken me nearly three years to figure out on my own. These days, I am an active participant in my local support group and always look forward to the in-person or online meetings in which I allow myself to be vulnerable in an extremely supportive and non-judgment environment.

As hard as it would have been, I should have disconnected from the on-line world. The support needed in those first few days after the diagnosis starts with your loving, caring and supportive family, friends or extended community support, in the real world.

I would have searched for one good reference book. Only one. For the past eight years, mine has been "Parkinson's Disease Treatment Guide for Physicians," by J. Eric Ahlskog. I still rely and refer to it from to time. It's the only one I read.

I would have avoided reading every article, link, case study, and alternative therapy at the very early stages of my journey. I realize now that I didn't have to be an expert on every aspect of Parkinson's disease within the first 24 hours.

I would have liked to have seen the neurologist within a few days or a week of receiving my diagnosis. This would have helped to get answers far sooner to all the initial questions that flooded into my head a few days after that life changing day.

For the first 90 days, I would have kept a detailed log on the timing of my medication and meals, noting and describing any side effects, and my body's reaction to the medication. I would have made a note of all the questions to ask and a list of topics to discuss.

One of the first discussion points would have been whether there was any benefit to defer initiating the drug therapy. My first neurologist didn't give me much time to discuss this. I was left to conducting my own research. What I found out from the very start was that the drugs, unfortunately, don't cure us. Once we have the disability, we've got it – until the cure is found.

With little or no physical symptoms of Parkinson's disease at the time of diagnosis, chances are that a discussion with the neurologist around diet and exercise would have take priority over any recommendation or implementation of drug therapy.

The optimal goal for taking the medication is to live a life, symptom free for as long as possible. I chose not to defer drug therapy. Professionally, as a lawyer, a tremor in my right hand at the time may have been misconstrued by a client as nervousness, lack of confidence, or simply could have caused a distraction to our discussions. Personally, I was very self conscious of my tremor in the early days and that contributed to my increased levels of anxiety.

To someone else, in a more active working environment, a slight tremor may not be bothersome at all. But it's also important to remember that employees have a duty to perform their job safely, which includes the need to understand their job and the impact that Parkinson's disease (or any other disability for that matter) could have on their safety and the safety of others.

It's really at the point when the physicality of the condition starts to interfere with social interactions or in the reduction of recreational activities that more serious consideration should be given to introducing drug therapy.

There is no evidence to suggest that deferring taking the drugs will result in a better response if taken later in the course of Parkinson's disease.[21] I understand this to mean that there is no sort of "pool of dopamine" that could be added to, and then withdrawn against when needed.

---

[21] Eric Ahlskog J.E. *Parkinson's Disease Treatment Guide for Physicians.* Oxford Press, 2009, p.106

Another discussion would have been on the side effects of long-term drug use. Dyskinesias is typically a side effect of long-term use of Sinemet (the combined carbidopa/levodopa tablet). It manifests as an involuntary movement of a body part, typically at the peak of the dosage. Nearly 100 percent of Young Onset Parkinson's disease patients below the age of 40 will develop dyskinesias after 5 years.[22] The good news is that this can be resolved with a dose reduction.

The bad news is that the dose reduction can result in the development of something

---

[22] Ahlskog, supra, pp. 108–109

else, dystonia. Dystonia is associated with dopamine deficiency. When I was considering a change to my dosage, my second neurologist recommended that, over two months, I keep a detailed record of the dosage and time of taking my drugs, and then record if and when I experienced any involuntary movements. That way, it was easier for him to decide if I was experiencing dyskinesia or dystonia and could then adjust the dosage accordingly.

Dr. Ahlskog concludes this subject with the following statement: "Maintain patients in the mainstream of their lives."[23]

---

[23] *Ahlskog, supra, p. 106*

It's a personal choice, ultimately. Your mainstream will differ from mine. But being more informed will allow for better decisions.

As if a diagnosis of Parkinson's disease, a chronic, progressive condition for which there is with no cure, isn't enough to deal with, add dementia into the mix and living with the disease gets scarier.

This daunting subject came up as a result of a second neuro assessment that I undertook recently.

My neurologist wanted to assess my cognitive functioning against my first assessment in 2018. Before the test I took some comfort in the statistics. In general, dementia seems to more frequently affect patients over the age of 70 and those in the late stages of the disease. My results showed mild cognitive impairment that concerned the neurologist, leading to a second diagnosis, "PD with mild cognitive impairment."

I initially felt like Bill Murray in "Groundhog Day." There I was, again getting another diagnosis, eight years after my first. I would have to share the news with my family, again. I would have to adopt and live with a new challenge, again.

But the big difference this time, was how I reacted to the news. I knew what I wouldn't do and knew what I should do. I was not going to repeat what I had done on the very first day of my diagnosis. I was going to avoid Google and YouTube.

Instead, I had my "toolkit" full of all the coping skills and strategies that I had researched and taught myself. I reacted to the news with a stronger mindset.

I was able to digest the topic less emotionally and with a calmer mind. I could stand back and observe the news as opposed to being overwhelmed and consumed by it. With a calmer mind, I again referenced Dr. Ahlskog's book, my one and only reference guide.

What I learned and tried to interpret from my non-medical perspective is that dementia associated with Parkinson's disease is a secondary dementia, meaning that it develops from a separate source. In contrast, dementia in Alzheimer's disease is a primary dementia, meaning that it doesn't result from any other disease. People with Alzheimer's disease face a progressive loss of intellectual and mental function. With Parkinson's disease however, having some cognitive impairment doesn't mean that the full-blown dementia is guaranteed. So, the good news is that the development of Alzheimer's does not automatically follow from having Parkinson's dementia.

Also, cognitive impairment may be the result of other causes or factors like medications, sleep disorders, depression, or brain lesions, some of which are treatable independently. All of these issues must be noted and shared with your primary health care provider.

Having adopted a different approach to the news shared by the neurologist, I was able have a more engaged discussion with my family and make better, less emotional, more rational decisions on my future course of treatment.

CHAPTER NINE
Through Sickness and Through Health

*"'Through sickness and through health' sounds so
simple on your wedding day, but in reality they become
significant words that are a huge responsibility and
show true character to navigate."*

- Yolanda Hadid

Now, ten years in with Parkinson's
disease, I have come to accept that there
won't be a return to a former routine.
Having to live with Parkinson's disease
everyday is the routine. And, although I have
the condition, the burden is shared by

Melissa. That too started on the day I was diagnosed.

She was waiting anxiously to hear from me after my appointment with the neurologist, and when I called her, she was driving home. She was so shocked to hear the news that she had to pull over to the side of the road to catch her breath and gather herself. Her mind was racing with thoughts of disbelief, helplessness and denial. She knew that our lives from that day forward would have to change, but she had no idea the extent of it and the challenges that I would face. But, one thing she did know was that our unconditional love for each other, our mutual respect and true-life partnership, was unshakable and unbreakable. It would sustain us.

Truth be told, without her I don't think I would have ever finished high school, qualified as a lawyer in three countries, or have been able to still enjoy a fulfilling, meaningful and rewarding life with Parkinson's disease.

The foundation of this strength and commitment lies in our marriage vows, particularly the one that refers to "through sickness and through health..." Sickness precedes health and it's sickness **and** in health, not **or** in health. I can think of two reasons why this is the case. First, a relationship is never tested in health. It's easy living at that stage, typically. But it is tested fundamentally, in sickness. The true value of the relationship can be measured in the darkest hours when facing a chronic or terminal illness, or another traumatic life changing event. Secondly, and unfortunately, there seems to be the expectation built in that sickness will form part of the relationship at some point.

In November 2018, I returned to South Africa with Melissa and our children. After spending a few weeks in Cape Town and then a few unforgettable days in the Kruger National Park, I surprised them by making a short detour to the same Phalaborwa

Commando Unit that I would have had to report to for my army training, had I not left for New Zealand. I jumped out of the SUV for a quick photograph, standing at attention, and saluting.

I was then, literally at the crossroads of my life. What would my life have become if I had completed my army training at that base? What kind of life would I have had in South Africa? Would I be happy? Would I still be living with Parkinson's disease?

These were some of the questions that I had in mind, but kept to myself, as we started driving to the airport on the last day of our trip to start the long haul back to

Canada. I savored the opportunity for us to be together again on another road trip.

As a younger father I always enjoyed our summer road trips. We often drove to Chicago to visit my brother and his family. Other trips took us to Michigan, Maryland, Florida and Minnesota for soccer tournaments and dance recitals. The best part was that the kids weren't buried in their own rooms, in front of the television, or playing video games. It was before cell phones, so we played music. Daniel loved "The Backstreet Boys" while Jenna knew every line, of every song, on every "Spice Girls" CD. We communicated with each other, not by typed texts, but with actual, spoken words. What a concept!

Glancing in the rear-view mirror from time to time, on that final road trip in South Africa, I realized how time flies. Car seats had been replaced with backpacks, "sippy cups" replaced with coffee mugs, and Daniel and Jenna had grown up into thoughtful and affectionate young adults. Each of them confident in making their own decisions and in the choices they had made in their respective partners, who we had invited to travel with us. Riding "shotgun," was my ever-present Melissa, who took the time to point out some landmarks and memories that she could recall from her own childhood as we sped along the way to the airport.

It had been a trip of a lifetime. I loved having the opportunity to introduce my family to some of my oldest and dearest friends and we spent a lot of quality time with my sister and her family. It was remarkable seeing cousins connect so deeply in just a matter of hours. I take comfort in knowing that those bonds will endure, despite the long distance and time separating them from each other.

Throughout the visit, I channeled a tour guide. I showed the kids where I had lived and the primary school that I had attended.

I took them to Clifton Beach where I had met Melissa all those years before. I introduced them to some of my favorite South African foods: biltong (beef jerky, but better), tomato flavoured chips (that's ketchup), and a real South Africa braai (BBQ) under glorious African cloudless blue skies, and warm, early summer temperatures.

I came to realize that I had one more thing in common with Micheal J. Fox. Like his character, "Marty McFly," in the movie "Back to the Future," I too had gone back to the future.

The last few hours of the drive flew by. Sensing that our trip was coming to an end, the headphones came off, cell phones were put down and the radio turned off. We just started talking and didn't stop. I rattled off the list of questions that I had kept to myself at the start of the drive, and was overwhelmed with some of the astute, profound and mature responses that I heard from my own children.

Back when I first learned my diagnosis, being at home during the day was a rare occurrence for me. Seeing me return home after my appointment with the neurologist concerned Daniel. He knew something was serious if I was home early. After sharing the news with him, the first emotion he recalled experiencing was fear. Fear of an unknown disease, fear for me and how I would cope living with it, and fear for himself and how his life would change as a result, too. That emotion then turned to anger. How could a person who had dedicated his whole life to the betterment of his family be plagued with such a life changing illness? It didn't seem fair to him.

Daniel expected changes to work routines, schedules, and roles and responsibilities within the family. But, what hasn't changed is the closeness of our relationship, the mutual respect that we have for each other and, first and foremost, my value to him as a father. He commented that my poise and grace living with Parkinson's disease has always had a positive impact on his life. To him, I displayed true bravery and courage. He saw me progress from struggling to even walk on the treadmill, to running half-marathons, enjoying listening to and playing music, and still being dedicated to him and to the well being of the family.

Like me, Jenna remembered a slight sense of relief when hearing the diagnosis. This balanced out the initial shock at the news. She had noticed that my tremors in my right hand were much more consistent and noticeable. She saw how traumatized I looked when I shared the news and saw right through my fake smile and timid reassurance that everything would be okay.

Once the medication stabilized my physical symptoms, it was easier for Jenna to forget what I had. Her friends were surprised when she told them that I had Parkinson's disease.

Jenna's first tattoo, just below her ankle bone of her right foot, is not the shape of a heart, or that of the Maple Leaf, it's the chemical compound of dopamine. To her, it's the outward manifestation of something that I lack internally. It's to remind her that what you see, is not always what you get; sometimes things from the outside looking in may be very different from the inside looking out.

As hard as it may be to see, Parkinson's disease has had a positive impact on my life. It presented an opportunity for me to re-invent myself emotionally and physically. It has given me the chance to forge deeper, more meaningful relationships with my family. But just as importantly, it has impacted the lives of Melissa, Daniel and Jenna in positive ways too, giving them clarity, purpose and value to their own lives, one day at a time.

I have a new sofa. I still have the old one, but I don't sit on it much these days. I do, however, find myself glancing at it when I head out for my morning run or on the way out to the gym. I didn't choose to have Parkinson's disease. I had no control over that development. But, what I finally learned was how to control my reaction to having it.

Parkinson's disease has taken my place on the sofa. It no longer controls or defines me.

CHAPTER TEN
Myths v. Facts

"The great enemy of the truth is very often not the lie, deliberate, contrived and dishonest, but the myth, persistent, persuasive and unrealistic."

- John F. Kennedy

We live in a 24-hour-wired-world. The accessibility to information, anytime, anywhere, can be daunting and overwhelming, and it becomes difficult to dispel the facts from the myths. These are mine:

Myth: PD is only found in older people.

Fact: PD can affect people as young as 30 or 40; however, the average age of onset is 60.

Myth: PD affects everyone the same way.

Fact: Everyone will experience the symptoms of the disease, and its progression differently. There is no one well defined course that the disease will follow.

Myth: PD is only a physical disease.

Fact: Often the diagnosis of PD is preceded by other non-motor symptoms like anxiety, depression and insomnia. In later stages, cognitive impairment may become another symptom to deal with.

Myth: PD causes uncontrolled, spontaneous movements.

Fact: The uncontrolled movement seen in many patients with PD is called dyskinesias. The disease itself does not cause dyskinesias. It is a side effect of the medication levodopa that is used to treat PD.

Myth: Dementia in PD will lead to Alzheimer's.

Fact: Dementia is a hallmark of Alzheimer's disease, whereas dementia may or may not occur in people with Parkinson's. There are some overlapping symptoms. But in general, Alzheimer's affects language and memory, while Parkinson's affects problem-solving (executive function), speed of thinking, memory and other cognitive functions, as well as mood.

Myth: The progression of PD cannot be stopped.

Fact: Although progressive, the incorporation of diet, exercise and the practice of mindfulness have been shown to effectively deal with the various underlying symptoms to maintain a good quality of life and slow its progression

Myth: PD is terminal.

Fact: Although progressive and chronic, PD is not a death sentence. When well maintained through a combination of medication, diet and exercise, many can continue to enjoy full and productive lives for many years into the future.

Myth: Genetics cause PD.

Fact: Recent research out of the Mayo Clinic does confirm a less than 5 percent genetic link, and more common when the onset occurs before the age of 30. It's a very small percentage of cases.

Myth: Being diagnosed with PD is the beginning of the end.

Fact: (Like me) many are living a life that, in many respects, continues to be fulfilling, meaningful and rewarding after being diagnosed.

CHAPTER ELEVEN
It's Okay to Laugh

"A day without laughter is a day wasted."

- Charlie Chaplin

I have a confession -- some of my best "one liners" or "zingers" are not original.

In the past, I have relied on Robin Williams, channeling some of his best comedic lines from the "Hellooooo...." in "Mrs. Doubtfire," to his "I'm sweating like some sort of farm animal!" in the "Birdcage;" from Rodney Dangerfield and his "I just can't get no respect," spiel, to Jerry Seinfeld's "Not, that there is anything wrong with that."

But nothing compares to the influence of John Cleese in the short but hilarious, "Fawlty Towers" television series and in the classic "Monty Python" movies.

The "Ministry of Silly Walks" is a sketch from the Monty Python comedy troupe's television show Monty Python's Flying Circus, which is entitled "Face the Press." The episode first aired on September 15, 1970. A shortened version of the sketch was performed for "Monty Python Live" at the Hollywood Bowl.

To me, this sketch encapsulates John's status as a comedic genius by combining the physicality of sketch comedy with well written and perfectly timed dialogue.

From time to time, I do experience "freezing." Many experience this motor symptom at some point during their journey with Parkinson's disease, too. When asked, I describe the feeling as a "brain hijack" to describe the experience of briefly stopping suddenly while walking or when initiating walking and being unable to move forward.

These days, when I freeze, I think of Cleese!

It tends to help me break the freeze and bring a smile to my face internalizing a little bit of John Cleese into my life with Parkinson's disease. I'd encourage you to watch the skit at https://www.youtube.com/watch?v=eCLp7zodUil&feature=youtu.be.

But more seriously, there are other techniques that are easier to adopt. The first thing to do when you feel yourself about to freeze is to stop, breathe and relax. Consciously stopping, even for a few seconds, may be all you need to do in order to break the "brain hijack." Other recommendations include taking a sidestep, marching on the spot, or counting out loud until you feel you can move forward again.

If you are listening to music through earphones, crank up the volume to your favourite song, and get your legs to move in step with the beat.

I cannot mimic the comedic genius of John Cleese's "Silly Walk." I don't have to because I have developed my own version. I have been known to walk backwards (pretending to be looking at something behind me). Oh, and if you see a 56-year old man in a suit skipping down the road in the financial district, that could be me!

Norman Cousins pioneered the idea of laughter as medical therapy. Cousins was an editor at the <u>Saturday Review</u> when he felt ill with a chronic inflammatory disorder characterized by crippling arthritis and severe pain. In his book,[24] he illustrates how, through laugh therapy, patient participation in conventional medicine, he healed himself and lived well into his 80s.

So, with that in mind, I present – [insert drum roll here]– my top ten "Perks of Parkinson's":

------

[24] *Norman Cousins, Anatomy of an Illness as Perceived by the Patient: Reflections on Healing and Regeneration*

1. My drinks are always shaken, never stirred.

2. Name of my new band - "The Movers & Shakers."

3. Some of my favourite songs - "Shake it Off" by Taylor Swift, "Shakey Ground" by The Temptations, or "Freeze Frame" by The J. Geils Band. Of course, don't forget "All Shook Up" by Elvis Presley.

4. Being the "shake before use" expert in and around the fridge around mealtimes.

5. The dedicated driver to the mall for the prime, designated parking spot.

6. Never having to buy an electric toothbrush again.

7. Performing "The Robot" dance move without too much practice required.

8. Airline priority boarding, even when seated in coach.

9. At drumming, the single roll drum rudiment easily becomes the double.

10. All my glasses of milk turn into milkshakes!

CHAPTER TWELVE
Quotes That Inspire

I have collected a number of quotes that have inspired me over the years. Some of my favourite are shared below.

"When you can't control what's happening, challenge yourself to control how you respond to what's happening. That's where your power is." — Unknown

"You either get bitter, or you get better. You either take what's been dealt to you and allow it to make you a better person or you allow it to tear you down. The choice does not belong to fate, it belongs to you." – Josh Shipp

"I believe that sometimes the bad times in our life put us on a direct path to the very best times in our life." – Unknown

"Live as if you were to die tomorrow. Learn as if you were to live forever." – Mahutma Gandhi

"Forget all the reasons it won't work and believe the one reason that it will." – Unknown

"Living mindfully is the art of living awake and ready to embrace the gift of the present moment." – Unknown

"In life, friendships change, divorces happen, people move on, others die. Money and jobs will come and go. Live long enough and your health and body will change. It goes with the territory of being human. The fact that you are still here gives you an advantage. Don't look back. Look straight ahead! Decide to use all of your knowledge, skills, experiences and your life lessons from your mistakes, defeats and setbacks, to start over again. Life changes. You may not have the same life as before, but you can still enjoy your life!" - Les Brown

"Life can still be beautiful, meaningful, fun, and fulfilling even if things don't turn out the way you planned." - Lori Deschene

"Sometimes the smallest step in the right direction ends up being the biggest step of your life. Tiptoe if you must, but take a step." - Naeem Callaway

"You fall, you rise, you make mistakes, you live, you learn. You're human, not perfect. You've been hurt, but you're alive. Think of what a precious privilege it is to be alive--to breathe, to think, to enjoy, and to chase the things you love. Sometimes there is sadness in our journey, but there is also lots of beauty. We must keep putting one foot in front of the other even when we hurt, for we will never know what is waiting for us just around the bend." - Unknown

"If you can't fly then run, if you can't run then walk, if you can't walk, then crawl, but whatever you do you have to keep moving forward." – Martin Luther King Jr.

"I've learned that everything happens for a reason, every event has a why and all adversity teaches us a lesson...Never regret your past. Accept it as the teacher that it is."
– Robin Sharma

Epilogue

As I reflected on the completion of my manuscript about my life with Parkinson's disease, I asked myself a question. Given the choice, would I have chosen to have it? Who would want to be diagnosed with a chronic, neurodegenerative illness, for which there is no cure? Who would want to experience a continuous tremor in one hand, and a dropped foot making walking difficult? Who would want to experience anxiety, depression and insomnia? Who would want to have cognitive impairment making communication difficult at times?

Over the past ten years I have experienced many of these symptoms, so I do feel that I have enough authority to have asked that question. And, as strange as it may seem, I concluded that I would have chosen to have it. Let me explain why.

From the outset, let me clarify that it would have been a lot easier to come to an opposite decision if my drug therapy had not been as effective as it has been over the majority of my ten year journey with Parkinson's disease. My motor symptoms have, generally, been well maintained. The incorporation of other lifestyle changes like running, cycling, drumming, boxing, and meditation have assisted me to deal with many of the non-motor symptoms positively, too.

Typically, as we all know, the average age for onset is 60. Being diagnosed at the age of 49 changed my perspective and relationship with time. I have had time to forge a deeper relationship with my wife. I have been able to be a father to my children. I have had the time to enjoy the company of my friends. I have had the time to laugh more deeply, and even, at times, to cry more often. I have come to appreciate life as it unfolds in the present, instead of ruminating on events of the past, or try to predict the future.

I have had the time to feel gratitude, be thankful and appreciate the simple things in life – the quiet of an early morning, the savour of the first sip of a cup of hot tea, the dawn of a new day, the calm sound of waves crashing onto a beach, and the solitude of a setting sun.

I have had time to forgive and to seek forgiveness from others.

I have seen the best in many, true genuine interest and concern for my well-being. I also have had the opportunity to teach and educate others that what you see is not always what you get: that tremors do not necessarily equate to nervousness and that slurred words should not be interpreted as drunkenness.

Ultimately, Parkinson's disease presented me with the time and the opportunity to reinvent myself physically and emotionally. That has brought a higher sense of meaning to my life. I have a clear purpose and that is to live my best and most authentic life with Parkinson's disease.

Resources

CANADA

- Grimes D, Fitzpatrick M, Gordon J, et al. Canadian guideline for Parkinson disease. CMAJ 2019. doi: 10.1503/cmaj.181504

- Parkinson Canada - www.parkinson.ca

- Regional Offices of Parkinson Society Canada also have their own websites and resources, including:

  - Parkinson Society British Columbia www.parkinson.bc.caParkinson

  - Society Saskatchewan www.parkinsonsaskatchewan.ca

  - Parkinson Society Central & Northern Ontario www.parkinsonCNO.ca

  - Parkinson Society Southwestern Ontario www.parkinsonsociety.ca

- Parkinson Society Eastern Ontario
  www.parkinsons.ca

- Parkinson Society Quebec
  www.parkinsonquebec.ca

- Parkinson Society Maritime Region
  www.parkinsonmaritimes.ca

- Parkinson Society Newfoundland and Labrador
  www.parkinsonnl.ca

- E-Parkinson Post: For Canadians Living with
  Parkinson's http://parkinsonpost.com

USA

- American Parkinson Disease Association
  www.apdaparkinson.org

- National Young Onset Center
  www.youngparkinsons.org

- Davis Phinney Foundation for Parkinson's
  http://www.davisphinneyfoundation.org/

- MedlinePlus http://www.nlm.nih.gov/medlineplus/

- Michael J Fox Foundation for Parkinson's Research https://www.michaeljfox.org

- National Institute of Neurologic Disorders & Stroke www.ninds.nih.gov

- National Parkinson Foundation www.parkinson.org

- Parkinson's Action Network www.parkinsonsaction.org

- Parkinson's Disease Foundation www.pdf.org/

OTHER

- Designing a Cure http://www.designingacure.com/

- European Parkinson's Disease Association http://www.epda.eu.com/en/

- Parkinson's UK http://www.parkinsons.org.uk/

- The Parkinson Hub http://www.theparkinsonhub.com/

- The Cure Parkinson's Trust http://www.cureparkinsons.org.uk/

- World Parkinson Congress
  http://www.worldpdcongress.org

- World Parkinson Disease Association
  http://www.wpda.org

Acknowledgements

First, and foremost, to my best friend and marriage partner for the past 33 years, Melissa, who gets an enormous amount of credit for sticking with me through thick and thin, through sickness and through health. To the world you may be Melissa, but to me, you are the world.

My two amazing children, Daniel and Jenna, who were both living at home when I was diagnosed. It has been an honour and privilege to be your father. I am immensely proud of the loving, mature and appreciative adults that you have both become.

To our beloved bichon-poodle, Becky who taught me that's it's okay to stare out the window waiting impatiently for the return of our pack leader. You will remain forever in our hearts.

To Joel and Eleanor, my two older siblings. Despite long distances separating us, thank you for always being a telephone call or text away. Older siblings have a special place in the world. They are both a link to the past, and a look into the future. Thank you for showing me both.

To my extended family, my parent-in-laws, sisters-in-law, nephews, nieces and friends, thanks for always being there for me, particularly during some of the darker days when I was first diagnosed.

Thank you to my career transition team who saw more success in my entrepreneurial future than me: Belinda Witzenhausen, Elizabeth Walford, Marguerite Senecal, Ron Chan and Kim Chernecki.

And my best and last thank you has to go to YOU - for buying this book, for reading it and adopting some or all of the strategies, tips and tools that I hope will help you live your best and most authentic life today.

About the Author

Larry Linton, B.A., LL.B, C.S., was progressing steadily through his career as a corporate immigration lawyer when he came face-to-face with a life altering diagnosis of Parkinson's disease in 2012. In his first book, Larry takes us on his life's journey before and after his diagnosis and how he reinvented himself emotionally and physically to live a life with Parkinson's disease that, in many respects, is more rewarding, fulfilling and meaningful after his diagnosis, than before. By sharing his life lived so far with Parkinson's disease and the coping skills that he has developed, Larry hopes to inspire others faced with a chronic illness or life changing event to live their best and most authentic lives, too.